INTERMI FASTING DIET PLAN

The step-by-step guide to boost metabolism healthy weight loss.

3 BOOK OF 12

By David Smith

Chapter 1. Intermittent Fasting Diet Plan and Metabolic Health

In the course of the last 10 to 15 years, intermittent fasting has arisen as an unpredictable way to deal with lessen body weight and improve metabolic wellbeing past basic calorie limitation. In this audit, we sum up discoveries identified with Ramadan and Sunnah fasting. We at that point talk about the part of caloric limitation as an intercession for weight control, yet critically, as a procedure for solid maturing and life span. At long last, we audit the four most normal intermittent fasting (IF) procedures used to date for weight the board and to improve cardio metabolic wellbeing. Weight reduction is regular after intermittent fasting yet doesn't have all the earmarks of being not quite the same as day by day caloric limitation when thought about straightforwardly. On the off chance that may likewise give extra cardio metabolic advantage, like insulin refinement, that is free from weight reduction. While no particular fasting routine stands apart as unrivaled as of now, there is for sure heterogeneity in reactions to these unique intermittent fasting eats less. This recommends that one dietary routine may not be obviously appropriate for each person. Future examinations ought to think about procedures for fitting dietary remedies, including intermittent fasting, in light of cutting edge phenotyping and genotyping before diet commencement.

1.1 Introduction

Physiological variations, like the metabolic adaptability to food accessibility and the need for energy stockpiling, were expected to endure intermittent food deficiencies all through human development. Stoutness gives off an impression of being the sign of modernization dependent on many contextual analyses archiving the variation of western ways of life. The exact worldly taking care of examples of our progenitors are obscure, however they were likely altogether different than the postindustrial upheaval taking care of examples portrayed by expanded feast recurrence and broadened eating spans with consumption moved to later in the day. Tragically, present day taking care of propensities regularly diverge from circadian physiology, which requires ecological signals (e.g., supper timing) to advance circadian synchrony. While circadian desynchronize has been connected to poor metabolic wellbeing and corpulence, feast timing has as of late been proposed to add to metabolic brokenness.

Intermittent fasting (IF) has arisen in the course of the last 10 to 15 years as an eccentric way to deal with conceivably decrease body weight and improve metabolic wellbeing past straightforward calorie restriction (CR). There are an assortment of intermittent fasting regimens with respect to feed and fast cycles, dinner timing, and energy consumption. Clinical preliminaries from the most widely recognized intermittent fasting regimens will be examined. These preliminaries share comparable qualities of delayed times of fasting. Alternate day fasting (ADF) and time restricted taking care of (TRF) are portrayed by broadening nighttime fasting. While ADF fuses a total quick every other day, TRF just abbreviates the day by day taking care of window. Both ADF and TRF may incidentally confine energy consumption and, hence, cause weight reduction. Interestingly, most alternate day adjusted fasting (ADMF) and 5:2 eating routine regimens use very low calorie consumes less calories happening irregularly all through a 7 d period. The degree that every one of these taking care of regimens influence all out body weight, body piece, and metabolic wellbeing are examined underneath.

1.2 Intermittent Fasting Diet Plans Help Boost Your Metabolism

Intermittent fasting is an eating design that includes times of food limitation (fasting) trailed by typical eating. This example of eating could assist you with getting thinner, diminish your danger of sickness and increment your life expectancy. A few specialists even case that its helpful consequences for digestion make it a better method to shed pounds than standard calorie limitation.

Intermittent fasting

Acetate
Lactate

Beiging

Metabolic improvements

Intermittent fasting is a basic, powerful way to deal with fat misfortune that is moderately simple to adhere to. Studies have shown that with regards to weight reduction, intermittent fasting can be similarly just about as viable as conventional calorie limitation, if not more.

Indeed, a 2014 survey tracked down that intermittent fasting could assist individuals with losing an amazing 3–8% of their body weight in 3 multi week. Besides, a new audit reasoned that in overweight and hefty individuals, intermittent fasting might be a preferable way to deal with weight reduction over exceptionally low calorie slims down.

Curiously, this way to deal with eating may likewise profit your digestion and metabolic wellbeing. There are a couple of various approaches to attempt intermittent fasting. A few group follow the 5:2 eating routine, which includes fasting for two days per week. Others practice substitute day fasting or the 16/8 strategy. On the off chance that you are keen on attempting intermittent fasting, you can peruse more about it in this itemized direct for fledglings.

Intermittent fasting is an incredible weight reduction instrument. It can likewise improve your digestion and metabolic wellbeing. Numerous individuals accept that skipping dinners will make your body adjust by bringing its metabolic rate down to save energy.

It's grounded that extremely significant stretches without food can cause a drop in digestion. Nonetheless, considers have shown that fasting for brief periods can really expand your digestion, not back it off. One investigation in 11 sound men tracked down that a 3 day quick really expanded their digestion by a noteworthy 14%. This expansion is believed to be because of the ascent in the chemical norepinephrine, which advances fat consuming. Fasting for brief periods can somewhat help your digestion. Be that as it may, fasting for extensive stretches may have the contrary impact.

Intermittent fasting decreases metabolism less than continuous calorie restriction. At the point when you get more fit, your metabolic rate goes down. Some portion of this is on the grounds that getting more fit causes muscle misfortune, and muscle tissue consumes calories nonstop.

In any case, the lessening in metabolic rate seen with weight reduction can't generally be clarified by the deficiency of bulk alone. Serious calorie limitation over an extensive stretch can make your metabolic rate drop, as your body enters supposed starvation mode (or "versatile thermogenesis"). Your body does this to moderate energy as a characteristic protection against starvation.

This has been shown significantly in an investigation of individuals who lost a lot of weight while taking an interest in the Biggest Loser show on TV. Members followed a calorie limited eating routine and serious exercise routine to lose a lot of weight.

The examination tracked down that six years after the fact, a large portion of them had recovered essentially the entirety of the weight they had lost. Nonetheless, their metabolic rates had not returned up and stayed around 500 calories lower than you would expect for their body size.

Different examinations researching the impacts of calorie limitation on weight reduction have discovered comparative outcomes. The drop in digestion because of weight reduction can add up to many calories each day.

This affirms that "starvation mode" is genuine and can halfway clarify why numerous individuals who shed pounds wind up recovering it. Given the momentary impacts of fasting on chemicals, it's conceivable that intermittent fasting may decrease the drop in metabolic rate brought about by long haul calorie limitation.

One little examination showed that getting in shape on another day fasting diet didn't decrease digestion more than 22 days. Be that as it may, as of now there is no quality exploration accessible taking a gander at the drawn out impacts of intermittent fasting abstains from food on metabolic rate. One little examination recommends that intermittent fasting may decrease the drop in metabolic rate that is related with weight reduction. More examination is required.

1.3 Intermittent Fasting and Different Religions

Numerous types of strict fasting can be found in Christianity, Judaism, and Islam. While explicit regimens change by length and dietary examples, numerous diets decrease creature protein, refined food sources, and different extravagances while advancing admission of products of the soil, expanded social commitment, and petition. Sunnah and

Ramadan, diets inside Islam, will be talked about as these methodologies bear similitudes to the common intermittent fasting approaches.

1.3.1 Ramadan Fasting

Muslims noticing Ramadan generally are not permitted to eat, drink, smoke, or participate in any erotic action among sunrise and dusk during the Holy month. It is a typical practice to wake right on time to eat before sunrise. Hence, energy admission is confined to evening, evening time, and early morning in a bimodal example. Concern has been brought in regards to this training up in those with diabetes. Here, we sum up the cardio metabolic impacts of Ramadan fasting inside the overall grownup populace.

Weight, Body Composition, and Energy Metabolism Changes

A few Meta analyses have detailed weight reduction following Ramadan fasting with starting weight record (BMI) decidedly corresponded with the size of weight reduction. Notwithstanding, complete weight recapture is frequently noticed 2 to 5 weeks after Ramadan. A few investigations have announced no adjustment of body weight, however two of these Meta analyses featured more articulated weight reduction in guys contrasted and females. Thinking about the positive relationship between the quantity of fasting days and the noticed size of weight reduction, blunted weight reduction is normal among females since fasting isn't permitted during monthly cycle. As regularly knowledgeable about weight reduction, enhancements in body arrangement like diminished fat mass and decreased midsection periphery are seen with Ramadan fasting. Diminishes in fat free mass are additionally noticed yet less significantly than fat mass. Besides, ongoing examinations report no impact of Ramadan fasting on resting metabolic rate or energy use, yet expanded fat oxidation and diminished starch oxidation have been accounted for.

Cardio metabolic health changes during Ramadan fasting

Meta analyses of Ramadan fasting have revealed cardio metabolic benefits among sound people with irregularities in regards to upgrades in lipid profiles. Detailed a slight abatement in complete cholesterol and fatty substances, a huge reduction in low density lipoprotein (LDL) cholesterol, and no adjustment of high density lipoprotein (HDL) cholesterol. Comparatively noted unassuming enhancements in fatty substances and detailed an expansion in HDL cholesterol. Remembered reads for competitors and pregnant ladies. They too detailed an expansion in HDL cholesterol, yet were the just analysis to report an increment in LDL cholesterol. All audits and Meta analyses propose sex specific impacts of Ramadan fasting, however they don't appear to concur. For instance, a subgroup examination shows bigger expansions in HDL cholesterol in females and more articulated abatements in fatty oils in guys. Alternately, other Meta analyses demonstrate an increment in HDL cholesterol in guys and a reduction in fatty oils in females. The justification such inconsistencies is obscure, however it could originate from an excessively higher male example and various standards utilized for study determination. Extra subgroup examinations demonstrate more prominent wellbeing enhancements comparative with pattern wellbeing, age, and decrease in body weight. Two Meta analyses revealed insignificant enhancements in fasting glucose among the two people. Until this point, it stays hazy how Ramadan fasting may decrease fasting insulin and improve insulin opposition. A few examinations have shown a decrease in insulin fixations and an improvement in insulin obstruction (homeostatic model appraisal of insulin opposition), while others report an increment in insulin and insulin opposition or no change by any means. Studies exploring the impact of Ramadan fasting on metabolic wellbeing utilizing more powerful methods, for example, the hyperinsulinemic euglycemic clip, are justified to additional logical comprehension of the impact of Ramadan fasting on metabolic wellbeing.

1.3.2 Sunnah Fasting

Sunnah fasting is rehearsed year round and remembers fasting week after week for Mondays and Thursdays with an extra 6 days of fasting in the Shawwal month. Two examinations by a similar exploration bunch surveyed 12 weeks of week after week Sunnah fasting joined with every day CR in more established guys from Malaysia. Sunnah fasting comprised of a little dinner preceding dawn and a full supper after nightfall; also, members were approached to limit calories by 300 to 500 kcal/d and to build admission of good food varieties. The two investigations demonstrated a general energy shortfall of 18% and weight reduction of 3%. Fat mass diminished by about 6% to 8%. While fat free mass was unaltered in one examination, another investigation showed a slight reduction that was not fundamentally not quite the same as the benchmark group. Just surveyed cardio metabolic results and noted reductions in both absolute cholesterol and LDL cholesterol by 8% and a diminishing in systolic and diastolic blood pressures by 4.5% and 2.6%, separately. There was no adjustment of glucose, and insulin was not announced.

Extra work by looked at whether as an accentuation on faith based dietary practices could advance wellbeing following Ramadan for 12 weeks. The benchmark group was relegated to standard dietary counsel, while the mediation bunch was additionally given faith based dietary guidance, for example, the incorporation of Sunnah fasting. The event of fasting twice week by week (Monday and Thursday) was unaltered; nonetheless, fasting once week by week (Monday or Thursday) expanded in the mediation bunch. There was no adjustment of fasting recurrence in the benchmark group. A decline in BMI from standard was seen in the mediation bunch, yet was not altogether unique in relation to the benchmark group. The mediation bunch likewise experienced humble upgrades in cardio metabolic wellbeing, for example, diminishes in diastolic circulatory strain and expansions in HDL cholesterol. Notwithstanding, this could likewise be a result of upgraded vegetable admission happening in the mediation bunch. Together, these examinations recommend that the act of Sunnah fasting may advance cardio metabolic wellbeing. A continuation of Ismail et al. on a bigger and more generalizable scale could have general wellbeing suggestions inside Muslim people group.

1.4 Intermittent Fasting improve Weight Management

In this segment, we survey the extraordinary IF procedures that have been read for weight the board, with included accentuation their cardio metabolic wellbeing sway. These incorporate the 5:2 eating regimen, ADF, ADMF, and TRF.

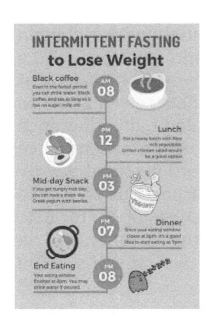

1.4.1 The 5:2 Intermittent Fasting Diet Plan

The 5:2 eating routine is a mainstream diet that imparts a few similitudes to Sunnah fasting, as the two regimens call for altered fasting to happen twice week after week. Until now, all 5:2 regimens have permitted 25% energy admission on the "quick day" as opposed to a total quick. This taking care of routine, joined with not obligatory benefiting from the excess 5 days, may inspire a week by week energy deficiency of 20 to 25%. Dinners devoured during the changed quick days are commonly eaten whenever. About portion of the preliminaries license members to choose two no consecutive quick days, while others require a more forceful methodology with back to back quick days.

Weight, body shape, appetite, and energy consumption changes

All 5:2 eating routine examinations have been planned as weight reduction intercessions, and a significant number of these investigations look at 5:2 versus day by day CR. Short term examines enduring 8 weeks have revealed high adherence to 5:2 weight control plans. In general adherence doesn't seem to contrast among 5:2 and day by day CR. Intercessions going from 4 to 24 weeks have detailed weight reduction of 4 to 8%. Weight reduction of in any event 5% is conceivable inside about two months. The adequacy of achieving in any event 5% weight reduction is comparable among 5:2 and day by day CR. Diminishes in fat mass regularly range from 9 to 13% with simply a 1 to 4% decrease in fat free mass and is like day by day CR. Members likewise report lower caloric admission during 5:2 contrasted with day by day CR. Diminished admission could be the consequence of transient ketosis, which may incompletely clarify the noticed concealment of craving evaluations and support of gauge ghrelin focus during 5:2 a chemical which generally increments with weight reduction and signs hunger. Introductory evaluations of yearning are higher during 5:2 contrasted with day by day CR yet seem, by all accounts, to be relieved by higher protein allow and standardize after some time. Further examination ought to interpret feed and quick day collaborations on yearning, totality, and satiation, while matching insights with biomarkers of craving.

Cardio metabolic health changes during 5:2 Diet Plan

Comparative weight reduction results make it conceivable to analyze weight loss independent cardio metabolic contrasts among 5:2 and day by day CR. Diminishes in absolute cholesterol, LDL cholesterol, and fatty substances as high as 13%, 15%, and 22%, separately, have been accounted for with 5:2. Humble upgrades in lipids are comparable among 5:2 and every day CR. The 5:2 eating regimen, in any case, seems to have an unrivaled insulin sensitizing sway. First noticed enhancements in insulin affectability following a half year of 5:2, which was marginally better compared to every day CR. Comparable discoveries were duplicated in two different examinations from similar agents. These perceptions could be clarified by the emotional expansion in insulin affectability quickly following 2 days of back to back fasting that waited all through the excess feed days. Moreover, differential adipokine reactions among 5:2 and every day CR could likewise assume a part. Among people with type 2 diabetes, decreased medicine use (i.e., insulin) and brought down hemoglobin A1C (HbA1c) were seen with 5:2, along these lines supporting the hypothesis that 5:2 advances insulin refinement. Future exploration should address whether pattern attributes can foresee which dietary intercession (5:2 versus day by day CR) is the best for an individual dependent on their metabolic wellbeing status.

Studies on weight loss maintenance and follow up during 5:2 Diet Plan

Following fruition of a 5:2 eating regimen, weight recapture is exceptionally factor and like day by day CR. Announced a 33% weight recover in returning members upon a 2 year follow up. In a similar report, HbA1c expanded, while complete cholesterol and LDL cholesterol got back to standard. Critically, different investigations diminished weight recapture while keeping up decreases in adiposity and cardio metabolic illness hazard through proceeded with commitment in weight reduction upkeep programs enduring 4 to 24 weeks. In examinations lacking kept advising, weight recapture happened and cardio metabolic hazard bounced back during follow ups enduring roughly a half year.

1.5 Alternate Day Modified Fasting and Alternate Day Fasting

Both ADF and ADMF switch back and forth between long periods of fasting and taking care of. Fasting days can go from 75 to 100% CR relying upon the fasting routine, and taking care of days are generally not obligatory. Fundamental work in this field used either a total quick (ADF) or a 20 hour quick every other day (ADMF). The inclusive daytime fasting has been concentrated less as often as possible because of helpless decency of a total quick every other day. Therefore, most ADMF conventions currently incorporate a solitary early afternoon dinner, which commonly falls inside a 2 hour taking care of window and allots 25% of energy prerequisites.

Changes in body composition, appetite and body weight during Alternate day fasting

ADF and ADMF preliminaries in people frequently bring about weight reduction either by plan or inadvertently, which is rather than mouse models exhibiting weight upkeep. Three short term preliminaries in male members were fruitful at keeping up body weight. Different preliminaries urged members to devour 145 to 200% of their energy needs on the feed days, yet members actually experienced accidental weight reduction. These reports recommend that ADF and ADMF regimens may have helpful worth as heftiness medicines. Mediations enduring 4 to about four months report weight reduction between 3 to 13%, while preliminaries stretching out to 24 weeks report weight reduction of 6 to 11%. Correlations of day by day CR against ADF and ADMF exhibit practically identical reductions in body weight and fat mass. Some of which report patterns for more noteworthy weight reduction during ADF or ADMF. Different irregularities exist. For instance, ADMF beat every day CR for weight reduction for the initial 4 months, yet not at ensuing time points reaching out to a half year. In different cases, ADMF inspired prevalent decreases in weight and fat mass contrasted with day by day CR. Similarly, there is no agreement as for fat free mass changes. A few no randomized preliminaries of ADMF propose fat free mass maintenance. This impact on fat free mass isn't rehashed across examines and is regularly the same contrasted with every day CR. Disparate ends could originate from differing levels of weight reduction, span of intercessions, and errors between body structure evaluation strategies (i.e., bioelectrical impedance versus dual energy X ray absorptiometry).

In spite of by and large high dietary adherence, for the most part great examination maintenance, and insignificant announced results, a few ADF or ADMF considers have detailed dropout rates more prominent than 20%. True to form, dropouts expanded when the span of the intercession was 12 weeks or more. It likewise stays muddled how well tolerated these kinds of IF eats less really are contrasted with every day CR, little examinations (20 members for every gathering) seem to report comparative dropout rates, while, bigger investigations (40 members) are ambiguous. These discoveries combined with inborn individual inconstancy in noticed weight reduction and the developing interest for exact clinical treatment, recommend that individualized weight reduction approaches might be advantageous. On the side of this, identification as a "major eater" was adversely connected with weight reduction probably because of the capacity to all the more likely make up for the quick day energy deficiency. There additionally gives off an impression of being differential reactions among segment bunches after pooling a few ADMF concentrates in an auxiliary investigation. Caucasians and more seasoned people experienced bigger weight reduction, which is steady with other day by day CR contemplates. Explanations behind these distinctions stay obscure, however both social and physiological underpinnings likely assume a part.

A group has investigated a few ADMF varieties that could expand worthiness and adherence. The standard ADMF approach takes into consideration just a solitary early afternoon dinner to be devoured on fasting days. Regularly, a low fat dietary example is suggested or given. This might be hard for calorie counters liking to eat later in the day or those wanting higher fat suppers. Inspected dinner timing and recurrence during ADMF and noticed no impact regarding weight reduction or changes in body organization when the quick day supper was given at various occasions or split into three little suppers. Furthermore, furnishing members with high fat suppers during ADMF likewise didn't prevent weight reduction. Other ADMF varieties have thought about whether weight reduction might be improved by fusing stimulating practices, like devouring higher dietary protein or including exercise. It is noticed that fat free mass maintenance from gauge with a high protein diet. Another investigation exhibited comparable decreases in body weight, fat mass, fat free mass, and instinctive adiposity between high protein varieties of ADMF and every day CR. Neither examination straightforwardly contrasted a high protein ADMF approach with a standard ADMF approach. There have been immediate correlations among ADMF and ADMF with work out. It is accounted for that the consideration of activity expanded weight and fat mass misfortune contrasted with ADMF alone. Essentially, detailed enhancements from gauge in body weight and body creation in both ADMF and ADMF with practice conditions, yet just the practicing ADMF bunch accomplished measurably higher fat mass misfortune from the control. Curiously, practice during ADMF seems to weaken dropout rates. This assortment of work assessing dietary and exercise varieties during ADMF focuses to the capacity to tailor ADMF as per singular inclinations and weight reduction objectives.

Hunger, which is generally an exploratory result, seems, by all accounts, to be controlled and may clarify the diminished reported caloric admission on feed days. Just one investigation contrasted hunger during ADMF with every day CR and announced no distinction between the eating regimens. Appetitive reactions to ADF or ADMF fluctuate by study and evaluation strategy. Three weeks of ADF improved day by day sensations of completion; yet, hunger remained. With ADMF, hunger sensations seem to die down after just fourteen days. This demonstrates that decency might be upgraded with the consideration of a little quick day feast contrasted and a total quick, yet this examination has not been made tentatively. Diminished sensations of appetite and expanded sensations of totality have likewise been seen after longer openness to ADF and ADMF intercessions (as long as 10 weeks). This proposes craving standardization with time. Reactions to normalized supper tests, addressing physiological hunger, have been conflicting across examines. It is accounted for no adjustment of ghrelin following 3 weeks of ADF. Then again, hunger was unaltered after 8 to 12 weeks of ADMF and a slight expansion in ghrelin was noticed. Discoveries identified with totality and peptide YY (PYY), a gut peptide which signals completion, are uncertain too. It noticed a moderate expansion in PYY (16%) combined with expanded sensations of totality (10%) after ADMF, yet it showed no adjustment of PYY or completion. ADMF and ADF may, accordingly, appease hunger over the long haul, yet the systems clarifying are muddled and conflicting.

Changes in cardio metabolic health during Alternate day fasting

ADF and ADMF effect by and large cardio metabolic wellbeing, however conflict exists when looking at explicit results. For instance, fasting glucose has been appeared to both increment (5%) and decline (2 to 5%) during ADMF while others show no adjustment of preliminaries enduring at any rate a month and a half. Moreover, fasting insulin may diminish 21 to 42% in examinations enduring 8 to 24 weeks, subsequently improving insulin opposition. Insulin affectability, then again, is unaltered when evaluated by means of intravenous glucose resilience test (IVGTT) and shows differential reactions to blended dinner resistance testing by sex. Because of a hyperinsuliemic euglycemic brace following two months of ADMF or day by day CR, detailed no distinction in insulin affectability. The impact of ADF on lipid focuses seems to rely upon sex and may require a more extended openness period to encounter benefits. A few examinations enduring at any rate two months have likewise shown aggregate enhancements in lipid profiles described by diminished fatty substances, LDL cholesterol, and absolute cholesterol. Advantages in all out lipid focuses are not all inclusive and may not be unique in relation to every day CR. Three investigations report no distinctions from every day CR for aggregate or LDL cholesterol after weight reduction, while another focuses to body weight free enhancements preferring ADMF. Critically, the improvement in the atherosclerotic profile of lipid particles appears to reliably improve, and introductory discoveries recommend it might beat day by day CR.

Reaction as per metabolic wellbeing status is maybe really convincing. A clinical preliminary in members with metabolic condition showed a more prominent diminishing in fasting glucose after ADMF contrasted with day by day CR, however no distinction in insulin opposition or fasting insulin focuses were noticed. Other auxiliary examinations give fundamental proof that ADMF might be more compelling than day by day CR for lessening diabetes hazard. Members with the most significant level of insulin opposition encountered the best improvement after ADMF. In an alternate examination of just insulin safe members, there were checked lessening after ADMF contrasted with day by day CR for fasting insulin (52% versus 14%, separately) and insulin obstruction (53% versus 17%, individually). Long term randomized clinical preliminaries are required in populaces with diabetes or pre diabetes to make explicit determinations in regards to sickness results after ADF or ADMF.

Studies on weight loss maintenance and follow up Alternate day fasting

Weight reduction upkeep following ADF and ADMF is sketchy. Until now, four examinations have assessed weight reduction upkeep all utilizing incomprehensibly various methodologies. Following two months of ADF or day by day CR, detailed huge weight recapture (30% of starting misfortune) in both eating regimen bunches during a 24 week unaided follow up period. Both eating regimen bunches kept up supreme misfortunes in fat and fat free mass. The corresponding tweaks, be that as it may, in percent fat mass and percent fat free mass were better with ADF contrasted with day by day CR.

This could be because of certain members keeping up ADF during the solo follow up. In the longest weight support correlation between ADMF (half CR on the quick day) and day by day CR, announced comparable weight recapture directions between every day CR and ADMF and no distinction in body creation. Curiously, people accomplishing at any rate 5% weight reduction, selected higher protein consumption all through the preliminary. Different investigations combined ADMF with day by day CR during the weight reduction stage while joining admission of higher dietary protein as a feature of the weight upkeep approach. Utilized high protein feast substitutions on feed (1000 kcal/d) and quick (600 kcal/d) days during weight reduction. During weight upkeep, a similar quick day dinner substitutions were utilized while the feed days decreased dependence on supper substitutions. Members experienced limited quantities of proceeded, yet genuinely immaterial, weight reduction (1 kg) more than 12 weeks of weight reduction upkeep. Cardio metabolic enhancements just arrived at importance after weight support, despite the fact that there was clinically huge weight reduction (5%) during the weight reduction stage. Contrasted ADMF with calorie restricted feed days with every day CR alone. Following the weight reduction stage, abstains from food similarly kept up weight reduction by following proposals for higher protein consumes less calories for an extra two months. Notwithstanding approach, way of life changes causing a supported energy shortfall are needed to accomplish effective weight reduction upkeep. Further examination is expected to decide if protein admission during ADF of ADMF impacts consistence, craving, or body arrangement.

1.6 Time Restricted Feeding

Rather than 5:2, ADF, and ADMF regimens, TRF doesn't deliberately force CR. Maybe, TRF expands the day by day fasting time frame by confining food admission to a decreased window of time. Until this point, many creature examines have revealed that TRF induces clear medical advantages, remembering decreases for body weight, food consumption, hyperlipidemia, ectopic fat, and markers of irritation, just as upgrades in heart wellbeing, malignancy results, and life expectancy expansion. Late TRF preliminaries in people have permitted a taking care of window between 4 to 12 hours, albeit a window of 10 hours is believed to be ideal dependent on glycogenolysis, unsaturated fat oxidation, and gluconeogenesis regulations happening without dietary glucose accessibility.

TIME
RESTRICTED
FEEDING

When should you be eating for optimal health?

Single arm TRF preliminaries have revealed 2 to 3% weight reduction more than 1 to 4 months. Gill and Panda enlisted 8 people with overweight and weight who detailed an eating span of more than 14 hour to pick a 10 hour not obligatory eating window of their decision for about four months. Critically, the members experienced weight reduction, diminished yearning around evening time, expanded in general energy levels, and improved rest fulfillment, which endured for 1 year after the intercession started. Another new examination enlisted more seasoned, inactive grownups with overweight and heftiness and confined their eating to 8 hour not obligatory adaptable taking care of window; study chips in likewise experienced huge weight decrease.

In more controlled preliminaries, eating prior in the day ("early TRF") or in the day ("early afternoon TRF") outflanked eating later in the day ("late TRF") for cardio metabolic wellbeing. It is conceivable that eating in synchronization with the normal circadian endocrine beat promptly in the first part of the day or around noon may hold the way to normally decrease energy consumption. In only 4 days, early TRF (8:00 AM – 2:00 PM) versus control (12 hour window: 8:00 AM – 8:00 PM) modified articulation in 6 out of 8 circadian qualities. This was joined by transient contrasts portrayed by a nighttime blunting of glucose evaluated by nonstop glucose observing alongside modified view of craving and internal heat level. Alongside this, there was a general lessening in hunger and expanded fat oxidation without affecting 24 hour energy consumption. A more drawn out 5 week hybrid preliminary in guys with overweight and pre diabetes announced that early TRF (8:00 AM – 2:00 PM) really improved insulin affectability by 24% and beta cell work by 13% when contrasted with a 12 hour energy coordinated with eating window (8:00 AM – 8:00 PM). There were additionally noteworthy decreases in pulse and oxidative pressure (8 Isoprostanes.) Directly looked at early TRF (8:00 AM – 5:00 PM) with late TRF (12:00 PM – 9:00 PM) in 15 overweight guys in a hybrid plan. TRF diminished body weight, plasma fatty substances, and postprandial glucose levels in the two gatherings, and a reduction in fasting glucose through constant glucose checking was noticed uniquely with early TRF. Late morning TRF approaches have detailed comparable upgrades in cardio metabolic wellbeing. For instance, a randomized controlled examination found that deferring breakfast and propelling supper by 1.5 hours each (or noontime TRF) for 10 weeks diminished muscle versus fat and energy consumption in an associate of for the most part female members. Another preliminary of early afternoon TRF (8 hour window: 10:00 AM – 6:00 PM) in 23 grownups with heftiness affirmed such enhancements in cardio metabolic wellbeing, including diminished body weight, energy consumption, and systolic pulse.

A couple of studies recommend that late TRF may deteriorate cardio metabolic wellbeing. Contrasted with devouring 3 dinners/d of an EU caloric eating regimen, burning through those equivalent calories inside a solitary 4 hour evening feast (1 supper/d) expanded systolic pulse, cholesterol, hunger, early daytime fasting glucose, just as postponed insulin reaction (by means of oral glucose resilience test). Nonetheless, one 8 week randomized controlled preliminary in 34 resistance trained competitors announced that late TRF (8 hour window: 1:00 – 9:00 PM) diminished fat mass while keeping up fat free mass, muscle territory, and greatest strength when contrasted with burning through similar calories across the whole day. This preliminary additionally set off a decrease in fatty substances, testosterone, insulin like development factor 1 (IGF 1), and interleukin 1 beta without any progressions in complete cholesterol or fasting glycemic markers.

1.6.1 Diet Plans of Time Restricted Eating

Is it conceivable to improve your wellbeing not by eating less, but rather by just shaving a couple of hours off your day by day eating window? A little yet encouraging new investigation recommends that limiting eating to 10 hours per day over a three month time frame can prompt weight reduction, a decrease in stomach fat, and enhancements in many danger factors that can prompt early demise. The examination, distributed in December 2019 in Cell Metabolism, included individuals determined to have metabolic disorder, a term for a few unique conditions without a moment's delay, including hypertension, high glucose, elevated cholesterol, and abundance stomach fat.

Despite the fact that analysts didn't specify what food sources or the number of calories to devour, members ate a normal of 8.6 percent less calories throughout the span of the three month time frame, and lost 3% of their body weight and 4 percent of their stomach fat. We are amped up for these outcomes, in huge part since time confined eating can be so broadly embraced in clinical practice.

Time limited eating is only one kind of intermittent fasting. Different alternatives incorporate 5:2 fasting, where you eat typically for five days and confine calories to 500 or 600 on the two different days, and substitute day fasting, where you limit calories to around 500 each and every other day.

A specialist doesn't really require additional preparation in diet or nourishment to prescribe time confined eating to patients. It's genuinely simple to disclose and for individuals to embrace. In this investigation we permitted individuals to pick their own 10 hour window for eating, which they had the option to incorporate into their every day schedule.

To perceive what effect eating for less hours daily would have on individuals with metabolic condition, examiners selected 19 individuals: 13 men and 6 ladies. Every one of the members participated in time limited eating; there was no fake treatment bunch. Most of the members were on a statin to diminish cholesterol, a medicine to decrease circulatory strain, or both. Before the investigation started, the normal eating window for the members was over 14 hours per day.

With time limited eating, you're just permitted to devour calories during specific hours. An ordinary window of eating time could be 8, 10, or even 12 hours.

In the fourteen day time frame before the examination started, scientists had the subjects record what and when they ate in a wellbeing application that can help track day by day eating, resting, and movement designs.

One strength of the examination was the granular data on the circumstance of eating it gave. It is outstanding at gauge [before the examination began] that numerous members were 'brushing' throughout the span of the day and part of the evening, with one member eating for 17 hours in a 24 hour time frame. This is likely a typical eating design in the United States today, she adds, and it can prompt abundance calorie utilization.

Every one of the members decided to start their 10 hour window between 8 a.m. what's more, 10 a.m., and end between 6 p.m. also, 8 p.m. Based on food utilization records gathered before the investigation started, specialists inferred that the members didn't skip breakfast, yet rather deferred it for a little while. The equivalent went for supper: Rather than avoiding the dinner, individuals ate their last feast before to oblige the timetable. At the point when they weren't eating, members were urged to drink water. Utilizing the wellbeing application, every individual logged what and when they ate, just as their dozing times.

There were no unfriendly occasions detailed. After the three month preliminary, not exclusively did the patients get in shape and fat, yet their "terrible" LDL cholesterol and circulatory strain dropped as well. Glucose and insulin levels started to improve also, showing better metabolic wellbeing.

The high hazard populace that this investigation included individuals with metabolic condition with gentle class one weight makes up a huge piece of the populace in the United States. As per the most recent information, more than a third of all adults in the United States meet the metabolic syndrome criteria.

1.7 Intermittent Fasting Provide Health Benefits Independent of Weight Loss

Our survey shows that intermittent fasting approaches may give medical advantages free of weight reduction. This is in concurrence with Meta analyses showing diminished fasting insulin, in spite of no distinction in weight reduction between intermittent fasting regimens and CR. It is conceivable that one intermittent fasting routine could beat another, yet this remaining parts to be straightforwardly tried. Besides, consistence to intermittent fasting and day by day CR is frequently equivalent and shows that one may not be better than the other to accomplish a negative energy balance. Regardless, rehashed models across each kind of intermittent fasting routine do demonstrate an insulin sharpening impact happening very quickly upon diet inception. It is conceivable that this intermittent fasting impact could be interceded through circadian science as diurnal varieties in glucose, energy use, and substrate usage favor eating prior in the day and fasting around evening time.

Significantly, the heterogeneity in the reaction to various intermittent fasting techniques recommends that customized approaches will improve weight reduction and upgrade cardio metabolic wellbeing. In this way, the following period of intermittent fasting exploration should tailor dietary remedies dependent on factors identified with a person's remarkable physiology, current wellbeing status, dietary inclinations, social impacts, and constructed conditions. This new section of exploration can possibly recognize ideal contender for a specific weight reduction treatment. Progressed phenotyping and genotyping to distinguish the subatomic transducers of dietary mediations may one day give the premise to better redo care.

Present day taking care of practices incorporate eating across expanded timeframes (15 hours) with the biggest extent of calories devoured in the evening. Proof from creature models presented to intermittent fasting demonstrate a circadian resetting impact that could counterbalance chronobiological desynchrony forced by 24 hour social orders. Then again, confounded food admission during intermittent fasting may add to such desynchrony. Proceeded with assessment of intermittent fasting can possibly explain the interchange between diet, digestion, and circadian physiology. Ramadan research gives understanding into postponed intermittent fasting in people as energy admission is limited to predominately evening hours and has been appeared to diminish rest and disturb circadian musicality. However our survey focuses to upgraded cardio metabolic wellbeing with Ramadan fasting. Restricting evening energy admission during reproduced night shift appears to counterbalance a portion of the cardio metabolic brokenness noted in night shift laborers. Such discoveries place that the metabolic impact of fasting may exceed that of circadian interruption. Accordingly, using intermittent fasting as a countermeasure to known and regularly unavoidable circadian disruptors, including rest limitation, social stream slack, and night shift, is a neglected space of interventional research requiring consideration.

1.8 Intermittent Fasting Aids in the Preservation of Muscle Mass

Muscle is metabolically dynamic tissue that helps keep your metabolic rate high. This assists you with consuming more calories, even very still. Sadly, the vast majority lose both fat and muscle when they get more fit.

It's been asserted that intermittent fasting could protect bulk better compared to calorie limitation because of its impact on fat copying chemicals. Specifically, the increment in human development chemical saw during fasting could help protect bulk, regardless of whether you're getting thinner.

A 2011 audit tracked down that intermittent fasting was more successful at holding muscle during weight reduction than a customary, low calorie diet. In any case, results have been blended. A later audit discovered intermittent fasting and constant calorie limitation to effect slender weight.

One ongoing investigation discovered no distinction between the slender weight of individuals who were fasting and individuals on consistent calorie limitation following two months. Nonetheless, at 24 weeks, those in the fasting bunch had lost less slender weight. Bigger and longer investigations are expected to see whether intermittent fasting is more compelling at safeguarding slender weight.

Intermittent fasting may help diminish the measure of muscle you lose when you get more fit. Nonetheless, the examination is blended. Despite the fact that examination has shown some encouraging discoveries, the impacts of intermittent fasting on digestion are as yet being explored.

Early examination proposes that transient diets support digestion as much as 14%, and a few investigations recommend that your bulk doesn't diminish much with intermittent fasting. On the off chance that this is valid, intermittent fasting has a few significant weight reduction benefits over abstains from food dependent on constant calorie limitation. By the day's end, intermittent fasting can be a profoundly compelling weight reduction device for some individuals.

Chapter 2. Intermittent Fasting Diet Plan and Type 2 Diabetes

Type 2 Diabetes is a metabolic problem described by hyperglycemia that causes various inconveniences with critical long haul grimness and mortality. The issue is fundamentally because of insulin opposition especially in liver, skeletal muscle, and fat tissue. In this audit, we detail the hormonal components prompting the improvement of diabetes and talk about whether intermittent fasting ought to be considered as another option, no restorative treatment alternative for patients with this issue.

2.1 Introduction

Type 2 Diabetes Mellitus (DM) is a typical metabolic issue portrayed by hyperglycemia brought about by different components including hindered insulin discharge, insulin opposition, diminished glucose usage, unreasonable hepatic glucose creation, and foundational poor quality irritation. As per the CDC, diabetes influences 34.2 million individuals in the United States (10.5% of the complete populace). Diabetes is known to be answerable for the improvement of different long haul difficulties, which add to the sickness' horribleness and mortality. For example, diabetes is the main source of renal disappointment, new beginning visual impairment, and no traumatic lower limit removal in the United States. The entanglements of diabetes can be either vascular or no vascular in nature. The vascular intricacies incorporate retinopathy, macular edema, mono and polyneuropathy, autonomic brokenness, nephropathy, coronary illness, fringe vascular infection and stroke. No vascular inconveniences incorporate issues with the gastrointestinal parcel (gastroparesis), changes in skin tone, expanded danger of contaminations, waterfalls, glaucoma, periodontal sickness, and hearing misfortune. At present the objective of treatment for type 2 diabetes is based on forestalling or postponing entanglements and keeping up personal satisfaction for the patient, as depicted by an agreement report for the administration of hyperglycemia by the American Diabetes Association (ADA) and European Association for the Study of Diabetes (EASD). While it is supported that patients with type 2 diabetes participate in way of life changes including expanded active work, weight reduction, and clinical sustenance treatment, a lion's share of patients require the utilization of drugs to accomplish control of their blood glucose levels. In spite of the fact that it has been very much portrayed that type 2 diabetes is a sickness of insulin obstruction, a lot of the clinical treatments that doctors use are based around the reason of giving the patient more insulin. For example, drugs like the sulfonylureas, GLP-1 agonists, DPP-4 inhibitors, and different insulin arrangements all work by either expanding the endogenous creation of insulin or expanding the measure of exogenous insulin got. While this attempts to diminish hyperglycemia in these patients, treating an illness of insulin opposition by expanding insulin might be counterproductive, prompting the necessity of expanding measures of prescription throughout an extensive stretch of time. Indeed, an examination showed that when treating type 2 diabetics with concentrated insulin treatment to accomplish tight glycemic control, the patients all created expanded hyperinsulinemia and weight acquire over a six month period.

Intermittent Fasting and Diabetes
What do the Dietitians Say?

Is it sustainable?

Is it safe?

Will I lose weight?

Will I be able to control my blood sugar?

Albeit the ADA and EASD portray the objective of treatment as being pointed toward forestalling or postponing the intricacies of this infection, the objective of this audit is to investigate the chance of utilizing intermittent fasting as a no restorative alternative for the treatment of type 2 diabetes through improved insulin affectability. While thinking about the restorative job of intermittent fasting in patients with diabetes, there are three chemicals that probably assume a huge part. These incorporate insulin, just as the adipokines leptin and adiponectin. It depict the impacts of these chemicals on different tissues. It is the motivation behind this audit to give knowledge into the impact of these chemicals on the advancement of insulin obstruction and type 2 diabetes, just as the advantageous impacts of intermittent fasting on these metabolic markers. Pushing ahead, we trust this audit is an outline of the current writing on the utilization and adequacy of intermittent fasting in the facility. We additionally trust this survey fills in as an impetus for doctors to distribute case reports and participate in controlled investigations with respect to intermittent fasting and diabetes.

2.2 What Method is used?
A writing survey was performed for articles identified with the effect of intermittent fasting on type 2 diabetes mellitus. Preliminaries were incorporated if the investigation configuration included one of the three most generally announced intermittent fasting regimens: substitute day fasting, intermittent fasting, or time confined taking care of. At last, considers were incorporated if the result estimates included estimation for fasting glucose, HbA1C, fasting insulin, leptin, or adiponectin both in patients with and without a background marked by diabetes. Rejection models comprised of copies, abstracts, no English articles, articles that did exclude human subjects, those that didn't report result measures for any of the

recently portrayed factors, and works that were unpublished or inconsequential to the subject of interest. Our underlying hunt returned a lot of examinations. Two analysts autonomously investigated modified works to decide if contemplates met our incorporation rules. Studies that met measures were then additionally evaluated to decide if they would be remembered for our survey.

2.3 Intermittent Fasting and Appetite Control in Type 2 Diabetics

Intermittent fasting has as of late acquired fame as a methods for improving body arrangement and metabolic wellbeing. Intermittent fasting alludes to eating designs based around the standard of devouring next to no to no calories for time frames going from twelve hoursq to a few days with a customary example. There are a few distinct regimens of intermittent fasting. One such routine is substitute day fasting, in which long periods of fasting are isolated by long periods of not obligatory food utilization. Another technique is occasional fasting, in which people (additionally alluded to as 5:2 or 6:1 fasting). At long last, the most known strategy is time limited taking care of, in which food utilization is just permitted during a predefined window of time every day, regularly with sixteen to 20 hours day by day diets.

Heftiness is known to be a significant danger factor for the improvement of type 2 DM. There are various systems accepted to add to the advancement of insulin obstruction in corpulent patients. These incorporate, yet are not restricted to, foundational ongoing irritation and ectopic lipid affidavit. Instinctive fat tissue is referred to work as both a paracrine and endocrine organ through the emission of adipokines. These adipokines are either proinflammatory prompting persistent low level irritation, for example, leptin, or mitigating, for example, adiponectin. Leptin is known to assume a part in the guideline of body weight through motioning to the nerve center and other cerebrum districts to stifle food admission and increment energy use. The fiery impacts of leptin are likely because of its part in the creation of IL-6, which prompts the amalgamation of C-responsive protein in the liver just as up regulation of the supportive of incendiary cytokine TNF-alpha. Curiously, patients with more elevated levels of BMI and insulin opposition were found to have expanded leptin levels, potentially meaning that patients with stoutness and insulin obstruction are creating leptin obstruction too. Despite what might be expected, adiponectin is known to have antidiabetic and calming impacts. Adiponectin follows up on different receptors that outcomes in an increment in skeletal muscle and hepatic unsaturated fat oxidation, decreased hepatic gluconeogenesis, and expanded glucose take up. It additionally applies mitigating impacts through direct activity on provocative cells, activity of NF-kB, and collaborations with TNF-alpha. Adiponectin levels decline with collection of instinctive with the aim of deciding degrees of leptin and adiponectin in patients with metabolic disorder. They tracked down that in patients with the metabolic disorder, which incorporates stoutness and insulin opposition, an irregularity in degrees of leptin and adiponectin seemed to assume a part in metabolic adjustment that expanded the danger of type 2 diabetes. Strangely, a few examinations have shown that intermittent fasting, even without fat misfortune, has brought about a decrease of leptin levels and an increment of adiponectin, which brings about upgrades of insulin opposition.

It has for quite some time been realized that limiting calories can lessen body weight and increment metabolic wellbeing. An investigation showed that 25% calorie decrease either through diet alone or diet related to practice prompted upgrades in insulin affectability and decrease in beta cell affectability in overweight, glucose lenient people. In any case, a few heftiness preliminaries have exhibited that people have huge trouble supporting every day calorie limitation for expanded timeframes. Then again, intermittent fasting has higher consistence and has shown guarantee in the improvement of metabolic danger factors, body arrangement, and weight reduction in fat people. It has been shown that these gainful impacts are expected to a limited extent to the shift during fasting from the use of glucose to unsaturated fats and ketones as the body's favored fuel source. During this progress the body starts to change from the combination and capacity of lipids to activation of fat as ketone bodies and free unsaturated fats. This progress of fuel source, or metabolic reinventing, has been featured as a likely component for a considerable lot of the helpful impacts of intermittent fasting. In conclusion, intermittent fasting has been appeared to diminish adiposity, especially instinctive fat and truncal fat, to a great extent because of gentle energy shortages. It is through this decrease in adiposity that patients may encounter enhancements in their leptin/adiponectin levels and affectability, prompting improved hunger control and lower levels of constant aggravation hence improving a few danger factors for type 2 diabetes.

2.4 Intermittent Fasting and Insulin Sensitivity

Insulin assumes a critical part in glucose homeostasis because of its impact in advancing the capacity and use of glucose. Notwithstanding, the impacts of insulin are not restricted to glucose homeostasis. Insulin likewise assumes a part in the incitement of DNA combination, RNA amalgamation, cell development and separation, amino corrosive convergence, protein union, restraint of protein debasement, and above all, the incitement of lipogenesis and hindrance of lipolysis.

It is the advancement of insulin obstruction, which is characterized as the need of higher coursing insulin levels to create a glucose bringing down reaction that is believed to be liable for the improvement of type 2 diabetes. To advance guideline of glucose homeostasis, insulin works essentially on receptors in skeletal muscle, liver, and white fat tissue. To put it plainly, there are a few proposed components in regards to the advancement of insulin obstruction. One of the more unmistakable speculations portrays the relationship of expanded adiposity and the resulting constant aggravation that prompts the improvement of insulin opposition in tissues.

Intermittent fasting, as depicted already, may decrease adiposity and in this way insulin obstruction by means of decrease of caloric admission just as because of metabolic reconstructing. What's more, energy/supplement consumption (like that accomplished through decreased caloric admission) has been appeared to advance better maturing and decrease in constant sickness through expanded enactment of AMP initiated protein kinase (AMPK). AMPK reacts to both to expanded AMP/ADP: ATP proportions just as to endocrine signs of yearning and satiety. The part of AMPK at a biochemical level is outside of the extent of this audit, anyway actuation of AMPK through a low energy state has been appeared to start physiologic reactions that advance sound maturing. Expanded degrees of insulin, regardless of whether through expanded energy admission or insulin obstruction, prompts the initiation of downstream middle people that at last restrain AMPK. The job of AMPK in improved insulin affectability is most apparent through the beneficial outcomes of the normally endorsed biguanide, metformin. Metformin is known to advance the enactment of AMPK, and has been demonstrated to be powerful in the therapy of type 2 diabetes just as in the alleviation of various persistent infection states. In principle, diminished energy admission, for example, that is accomplished through intermittent fasting, will prompt delayed diminished degrees of insulin creation and expanded degrees of AMPK, which probably assumes a part in the upgrades in insulin affectability and glucose homeostasis.

2.5 Intermittent fasting Role in the Treatment of Type 2 Diabetes

A few investigations have shown guarantee for the utilization of intermittent fasting conventions as a likely treatment for diabetes. Tables 1 and 2 outline the discoveries of a few late examinations with respect to intermittent fasting and its impact on measures including body weight, fasting glucose, fasting insulin, adiponectin, and leptin. The consideration/rejection rules can be found in the advantageous record. In a methodical survey and Meta examination that included investigations assessing patients both with and without pre diabetes (diabetic patients were barred), it was discovered that of 8 examinations looking at the impacts of an intermittent fasting diet to a benchmark group, BMI diminished. Moreover, of 8 examinations contrasting intermittent fasting with a benchmark group in the assessment of glycemic control, it was tracked down that the intermittent fasting bunch had huge decreases in fasting glucose levels. Finally, when contrasting leptin and adiponectin levels between the intermittent fasting subjects and the control subjects in all examinations, the commentators discovered expanded adiponectin levels and diminished leptin. Followed three patients with type 2 diabetes more than a while subsequent to starting intermittent fasting routine comprising of hours diets each week. Throughout the span of the investigation, all patients had huge decreases in HbA1C, weight reduction, and the entirety of the patients had the option to stop their insulin treatment inside multi month. Curiously, the three patients for this situation arrangement all detailed enduring fasting quite well, and no tolerant halted the intercession anytime out of decision. This proposes that intermittent fasting may not exclusively be effective as a no restorative treatment choice for patients with type 2 diabetes, yet upholds the idea that this intercession is average also. Played out a clinical preliminary in which grownups with type 2 diabetes were isolated into two gatherings, one discontinuous energy limitation and ordinary eating routine each and every other day) and a constant energy limitation bunch. After whole year of mediation, the two gatherings showed comparable decreases in HbA1C levels and more noteworthy decreases in weight in the discontinuous energy limitation bunch. At long last, a comparative clinical preliminary analyzed another day fasting routine (25% of energy needs on fasting days, 125% of energy needs on no fasting days) to persistent energy limitation (75% of energy needs every day) and a benchmark group of stout, .no diabetic patients. Over an intercession time of a year, there were comparative decreases in body weight, BMI, and fat mass between the other day fasting and constant energy limitation gatherings, anyway there were critical decreases in fasting insulin levels and homeostatic model evaluation of insulin obstruction levels in the other day fasting bunch. HOMA is a marker used to gauge levels of insulin obstruction.

2.6 Recommendations for prescribing intermittent fasting in practice

While substitute day fasting and occasional fasting have exhibited viability in improving metabolic danger factors, it could be hard to persuade patients to surrender or seriously limit calories for a whole one day period. In America, we regularly eat 3 suppers each day notwithstanding successive nibbling. Besides, in American culture most friendly commitment include food. Requesting that patients kill these encounters from their everyday lives may get troublesome, and in this way obstruct patient consistence. At last, patients changing to intermittent fasting routine may at first experience indications like appetite and crabbiness, albeit these side effects frequently scatter inside the first one month. In this manner, it would be more suitable to slowly present intermittent fasting as time confined taking care of. For instance, clinicians may initially prescribe that patients confine their admission to a day by day twelve hours period, ordinarily a short term quick. As patients become more OK with this example of eating, the taking care of window can be limited further. This permits the patient some every day adaptability in picking when to devour calories, accordingly improving the probability of consistence. In conclusion, patients who have gotten adjusted to time limited taking care of may decide to change to substitute day or intermittent fasting with the management and direction of an enlisted dietician. See Fig. 5 for an itemized illustration of an intermittent fasting solution.

2.7 Considerations while prescribing intermittent fasting in practice

While thinking about the utilization of fasting in patients with diabetes, various focuses ought to be gauged. In the first place, it is critical to talk about potential dangers related with fasting. Patients taking insulin or sulfonylurea meds ought to be firmly checked by their medical services supplier to forestall hypoglycemic occasions. Since considers are showing a diminished requirement for insulin in patients who follow intermittent fasting conventions, blood glucose levels and drug titration ought to be noticed intently by the doctor. Doctors should help patients make fitting acclimations to their prescriptions, particularly on long stretches of fasting. Doctors may decide to have patients keep day by day glucose and weight logs and send them week after week or fortnightly by means of electronic message to help suppliers in medicine titration after some time. Of note, while the objective of adjusting this example of eating is to lessen or dispense with the requirement for prescriptions, including insulin, there are circumstances in which insulin might be important, like extreme hyperglycemia. Inability to do so may bring about huge outcomes, for example, the advancement of hyperosmolar hyperglycemic condition. Extra concerns, albeit improbable, incorporate nutrient and mineral inadequacies and protein hunger. Patients ought to be instructed with respect to the significance of burning through supplement rich dinners and sufficient protein consumption during taking care of periods. Besides, it could be imperative to consider nutrient or mineral supplementation relying upon the patient's dietary practices and the ideal length of a fasting routine. Patients ought to likewise be guided on the requirement for satisfactory hydration during times of fasting, as they will be needed to supplant liquids that may typically be devoured through food notwithstanding normal every day prerequisites. As numerous doctors may not be prepared broadly in dietary sciences, and further, might not have the opportunity to follow day by day with patients to guarantee suitable healthful admission, discussion with an enrolled dietitian is energetically suggested. In conclusion, it is imperative to consider populaces in whom fasting may not be fitting. These incorporate pregnant/lactating ladies, grownups of cutting edge age, people with immunodeficiency, and people with hypoglycemic occasions, and patients who experience the ill effects of dietary problems.

2.8 Future research and Limitations

This audit is certifiably not a deliberate survey and as such does not have the ability to sum up all path with factual importance. Having said that, we featured the exploration that has been done in people and introduced proof that intermittent fasting improves insulin affectability, likely through a mix of weight reduction and "metabolic reinventing". There is a lot of exploration that has been done on the impacts of intermittent fasting concerning enhancements in body arrangement and metabolic wellbeing, anyway a lion's share of the information to date has come from creature contemplates, which were excluded from this survey. Despite the fact that there are various case reports showing critical upgrades in diabetic patients' glucose control, large numbers of the randomized controlled preliminaries neglect to incorporate patients with diabetes. This is a territory where further examination is required, as the current preliminaries (and case reports) remembered for this audit that have been done on diabetic patients have shown guarantee in improving metabolic wellbeing with almost no antagonistic impacts. Most patients doing some type of intermittent fasting experience gentle energy deficiencies and weight reduction that may not be suitable for all patients. Thusly, there should be more investigation into outlining the metabolic upgrades of intermittent fasting from weight reduction.

Type 2 diabetes distresses 34.2 million individuals in the United States, and is related with huge horribleness and mortality. Despite the fact that diabetes is portrayed as a turmoil of insulin obstruction, a lion's share of the drug medicines for this illness advance expansions in insulin levels to accomplish better glycemic control. This prompts various issues including weight acquire, demolished insulin opposition, expanded degrees of leptin, and diminished degrees of adiponectin. Intermittent fasting has become an inexorably known dietary practice for the improvement of body structure and metabolic wellbeing. It likewise has shown guarantee in the treatment of type 2 diabetes. This might be because of its consequences for weight reduction, as well as diminishing insulin opposition and an ideal change in the degrees of leptin and adiponectin. Patients may move toward their doctors with questions in regards to the execution of intermittent fasting. Also, doctors ought to know about the advantages of this dietary practice as a treatment for type 2 diabetes with the goal that they might have the option to help patients utilize this to battle the movement of their sickness.

2.9 Intermittent Fasting in Diabetes Mellitus Patients: Clinical Management

Intermittent fasting is expanding in notoriety as a methods for getting in shape and controlling persistent disease. Patients with diabetes mellitus, the two kinds 1 and 2, include about 10% of the populace in the United States and would probably be pulled in to follow one of the numerous strategies for intermittent fasting. Studies on the security and advantages of intermittent fasting with diabetes are exceptionally restricted however, and wellbeing suggestions shockingly today emerge principally from weight reduction masters and creature contemplates. Clinical rules on the most proficient method to oversee restorative intermittent fasting in patients with diabetes are nonexistent. The proof to assemble a particularly clinical rule for individuals with a diabetes determination is practically nonexistent, with only one randomized preliminary and a few case reports. This article gives an outline of the accessible information and a survey of the exceptionally restricted relevant writing on the impacts of intermittent fasting among individuals with diabetes. It additionally assesses the known wellbeing and viability issues encompassing medicines for diabetes in the fasting state. In light of those restricted information and an information on accepted procedures, this paper proposes master put together rules with respect to how to deal with a patient with either type 1 or 2 diabetes who is keen on intermittent fasting. The security of each significant drug treatment during a fasting period is thought of. At the point when done under the oversight of the patient's medical services supplier, and with fitting individual glucose observing, intermittent fasting can be securely embraced in patients with diabetes.

The term intermittent fasting implies diminished caloric admission on a discontinuous premise.

This can differ from a few hours during the day to a total 24 h period. It tends to be accomplished for strict reasons, for example, during Ramadan or Yom Kippur, or for wellbeing reasons, including weight reduction. In this article, we will address just non strict intermittent fasting directed for wellbeing purposes and will audit the advantages, either potential or demonstrated, just as security worries in patients with diabetes mellitus, the two kinds 1 and 2. Articles have been composed on the most proficient method to oversee strict fasting and the per user inspired by this subject is alluded to these articles

The term intermittent fasting, when utilized for wellbeing reasons or weight reduction, has been utilized to portray different sorts of caloric limitation. A few creators use it when a patient retains caloric admission for a few sequential hours during the day (regularly 16 h with all energy consumption during the other 8 h of the day), others for an entire day more than once per week, and others three or four days of the week. A few conventions permit protein consumption yet no carbs and still name it intermittent fasting. Others permit carbs or large scale/miniature supplements up to a furthest reaches that will in any case advance ketosis and, despite the fact that it is just a low calorie diet, because of the prevalence of fasting this has been named an eating regimen that imitates fasting. In all cases, no caloric liquid admission is allowed (which is one of the fundamental contrasts when contrasted with strict fasting) and thusly essentially decreases the danger of drying out and hypotension, a conspicuous thought in strict fasting.

2.9.1 How it Work?

Most investigations of intermittent fasting have zeroed in on weight reduction as the essential objective. Those investigations were led under the idea that the essential medical advantage of intermittent fasting emerges from weight reduction. Along these lines, the time confined taking care of, substitute day fasting, and 5:2 eating routine regimens are not planned to be ketotic, however to essentially actuate upgrades in wellbeing through the average components related with weight reduction. For a more intensive audit of human investigations of the impact of intermittent fasting on changes in weight.

While ketosis is neither an objective nor an assumption for those supper timing plans, some fasting regimens may accomplish ketosis. Somebody have utilized the expression "metabolic switch" to portray "the body's special shift from use of glucose from glycogenolysis to unsaturated fats and unsaturated fat inferred ketones". They bring up that "ketones are the favored fuel for both the cerebrum and body during times of fasting and expanded exercise".

The metabolic switch happens when glycogen stores in the liver are exhausted, for the most part 12 h after the suspension of food admission, and fat tissue lipolysis increments to create more unsaturated fats and glycerol. The free unsaturated fats are shipped to the liver where they are oxidized to beta hydroxybutyrate and acetoacetate. They are changed over to energy through beta oxidation. By and large, this cycle includes expanded coursing unsaturated fats and different changes identified with glucose and unsaturated fat digestion, whose changes were as of late detailed among people during water just fasting.

Peroxisome proliferator initiated receptor alpha incites the statement of qualities that intervene unsaturated fat oxidation in muscle cells. Curiously, insulin opposition delays the time it takes to flip the metabolic switch and along these lines among individuals with diabetes it might take more time to start utilizing unsaturated fats for energy. The entirety of the ramifications of this distinction are not seen yet conceivably have suggestions for the board of individuals with diabetes who participate in intermittent fasting, however this requires examination in individuals with diabetes.

In those regimens that don't include genuine fasting, the "metabolic switch" component would not draw in and apparently the system of activity is essentially diminished caloric admission. Other expected instruments of medical advantages from fasting are under examination presently. These remember the expected effect of intermittent fasting for aggravation, receptive oxygen species, circulatory strain, and cholesterol levels, a portion of whose changes may happen just because of weight reduction yet that may conceivably likewise be affected through instruments that are free of weight change. They likewise may remember an effect for the human micro biome, the human development chemical/insulin like development factor 1 pivot, mitochondriogenesis, invulnerable framework productivity, and autophagy. Autophagy directs the amino corrosive inventory, and this was as of late answered to be controlled in explicit examples during water just fasting in people. Beforehand, an example of expanded oxygen helping limit through higher erythrocyte tally and hemoglobin levels during water just fasting was accounted for that may improve metabolic working or abatement insulin obstruction. Different systems may likewise exist that are simply starting to be investigated. Further assessment of the components of conceivable wellbeing impacts of intermittent fasting in people is expected to completely comprehend the effect that it has on human wellbeing.

2.9.2 Benefits of Clinical Management

Insulin obstruction, the most unmistakable element of type 2 diabetes, has for some time been known to improve with caloric limitation. After a time of fasting, insulin affectability rises and insulin levels fall. These outcome in improved fasting and postprandial glucose levels. Furthermore, as insulin incites fat tissue development, there is less inclination to weight acquire and conceivably even weight reduction.

Intermittent fasting would thus be able to be required to impact weight reduction, particularly when it is led regularly. From the get go in the investigation of fasting's wellbeing impacts it was guessed that fasting could improve a portion of the significant bothersome impacts of weight reduction slims down. Intermittent fasting has now been appeared, in any case, in different little and momentary investigations to be correspondingly powerful as every day calorie limitation in delivering weight reduction. Along these lines, when done as often as sufficiently possible, fasting can be one alternative for sound weight reduction, however the best proof shows that fasting is certifiably not an unrivaled weight reduction technique.

Insulin obstruction is related with an expanded fiery state including raised C-responsive protein, diminished adiponectin, lower low thickness lipoprotein (LDL) molecule size, and other metabolic elements that all add to or are related with atherosclerosis and improvement of coronary course infection.

Besides, insulin is referred to be both atherogenic just as increment the danger of liquid maintenance and congestive cardiovascular breakdown. Subsequently, decreasing insulin levels through intermittent fasting would have the potential for diminishing major antagonistic cardiovascular occasions. Such decrease in insulin might be attainable. Written about three patients who had the option to suspend insulin treatment 5–18 days in the wake of starting intermittent fasting, during which they had supper however skipped breakfast and lunch on either substitute days or 3 days out of every week. Further examination of this speculation in bigger populaces is required, yet this finding is an enticing and possibly outlook changing outcome in the event that it tends to be securely and dependably rehashed in enormous populaces.

Intermittent fasting and calorie limitation have been appeared to improve different metabolic and fiery pathways. Included are expanded warmth stun protein, advancing cell autophagy, diminishing progressed glycation final results, expanded adiponectin, and diminished aggravation cytokines. Every one of these impacts bring about diminished vascular brokenness and would consequently be required to improve cardiovascular danger as well as mortality. Regardless of whether indeed the progressions because of fasting are critical and supported enough to do so stays to be demonstrated.

While there are no imminent clinical preliminaries of cardiovascular advantages from intermittent fasting (i.e., its impacts on clinical major unfriendly cardiovascular occasions), observational populace examines have shown cardiovascular and metabolic advantages a lower hazard of coronary course illness and lower hazard of diabetes from just one day out of each long stretch of energy limitation through fasting (rehearsed over a time of many years). One planned clinical preliminary did as of late report an impact of intermittent fasting on the control of hemoglobin A1C. Among a populace of 97 individuals with type 2 diabetes mellitus (40 of the 137 took a crack at the preliminary pulled out right on time), hemoglobin A1C decrease because of intermittent fasting was non subpar compared to persistent energy limitation. Sadly, weight reduction in that preliminary was not diverse in the fasting arm contrasted with caloric limitation, and other metabolic measures were not extraordinary. Generally, audits of the proof show that deficient human information exist as of now to suggest the utilization of intermittent fasting or low calorie diets to forestall diabetes or, among individuals with diabetes, to forestall its sequel.

2.9.3 Risk Factors

The most impending danger with intermittent fasting is the potential for hypoglycemia in patients who are on ant diabetic drugs that are related with hypoglycemia, explicitly insulin (both prandial and basal) and sulfonylureas (counting the short acting meglitinides). Any remaining ant diabetic prescriptions when utilized either as mono therapy or in mix treatment without insulin or sulfonylureas are infrequently, however not never, related with hypoglycemia, and the danger is in this way significantly less however still a thought.

With long haul intermittent fasting, one requirements to likewise be worried about protein ailing health if patients are not conscious to keep up satisfactory protein admission on those occasions when they are eating. Nutrient and mineral lack of healthy sustenance could likewise happen and, contingent upon how long seven days the patient is fasting and what they are eating when they do eat, might require taking nutrient as well as mineral enhancements.

Different dangers incorporate an assortment of potential damages identified with deficient energy admission and some because of lack of hydration. These incorporate wellbeing occasions that may happen among any individual who takes part in intermittent fasting, whether or not they have diabetes. Such unfavorable occasions may incorporate discombobulating, queasiness, a sleeping disorder, syncope, falls, headache migraine, shortcoming that limits day by day exercises, and exorbitant cravings for food. The presence of a constant illness, including diabetes, may expand the danger of encountering a significant number of these antagonistic occasions, as may different sicknesses including coronary vein infection, shaky angina, cardiovascular breakdown, atrial fibrillation, earlier myocardial dead tissue, earlier stroke or transient ischemic assault, most malignant growths, ongoing obstructive aspiratory infection, pneumonic embolism, asthma, fringe vascular thromboembolism, persistent kidney infection, and possibly different conditions. For individuals with these persistent sicknesses, little is thought about the reaction to fasting, in this way it isn't really that they ought not to take part in fasting, however that how their dangers because of fasting are changed is dubious and expect studies to be led in these populaces where raised wellbeing hazards exist. Positively, presenting such people to genuine unfriendly occasions like new myocardial dead tissue, stroke, or passing is unjustifiable and alert is the key as of now given the absence of proof in these populaces.

For conditions where drying out is a danger, like stroke, consolation to hydrate well during any fasting routine is suggested. Drinking water, including to supplant liquids that regularly would be devoured in food sources, is a significant thought for individuals of any age who are partaking in intermittent fasting.

Moreover, a few populaces have exceptional dangers and ought to be discouraged from taking part in intermittent fasting, particularly on the off chance that they have diabetes. This incorporates pregnant and lactating ladies, small kids, grownups of cutting edge age, and more established grownups who are delicate. People with immune deficiencies, including the individuals who have had a strong organ relocate and are on clinical immunosuppression, ought to likewise shun fasting. Individuals with dietary issues and those with dementia have special difficulties that will probably be exacerbated by purposely captivating in fasting, subsequently they ought not to follow intermittent fasting regimens. Patients who have a background marked by awful mind injury or post concussive condition may likewise be at higher danger of antagonistic occasions, and their necessities ought to be viewed as cautiously dependent upon the situation before starting a fasting routine.

2.9.4 Management
Patients with diabetes who are keen on intermittent fasting ought to be urged to take part in fasting with direction from a medical services professional, including doctors, nurture experts, doctors' aides, ensured diabetes

teachers, or enlisted dietitians. Explicit consideration ought to be paid to three contemplations: prescription change, recurrence of glucose checking, and liquid admission. The majority of these proposals depend on the clinical experience of the creators when there is no free writing, while a portion of the suggestions depend on distributed methodologies in investigations of intermittent fasting among individuals with diabetes.

2.9.5 Glucose Monitoring

Except if the patient is utilizing a sulfonylurea or insulin, the danger of hypoglycemia is low and no extra glucose checking would be regularly suggested during fasting. The patient ought to, nonetheless, be helped about the side effects to remember hypoglycemia and ought to be urged to check their blood glucose if any of the indications do create. A few patients will create manifestations reminiscent of hypoglycemia even with a blood glucose over 70 mg/dL, hence alert is demonstrated in the way to deal with their reaction to indications related to glucose checking.

In patients on a sulfonylurea or insulin (either alone or in mix with some other ant diabetic medicine), the danger of hypoglycemia is huge, and the patient ought to be urged to accomplish more regular blood glucose testing, particularly when initially beginning with intermittent fasting. Contingent upon the danger of hypoglycemia as surveyed by the expert, the testing could be as frequently as at regular intervals in the patient on insulin or like clockwork on sulfonylureas. On the off chance that the fasting is a 24 h or longer quick, particularly a water just quick, explicit thoughtfulness regarding the following daytime's fasting blood glucose perusing ought to be made.

Patients on insulin who will embrace intermittent fasting may be urged to utilize individual ceaseless glucose observing frameworks. On account of the framework, this would consider a hypoglycemia alert. With the Freestyle framework, while there is no hypoglycemia ready, continuous testing should be possible without extra cost or distress. The danger of hypoglycemia with intermittent fasting while at the same time utilizing insulin can't be over underscored and may even increment if the patient is effective in getting more fit because of the discontinuous quick. While depending on finger stick glucose testing might be satisfactory, having a nonstop glucose observing framework would by and large urge the patient to accomplish more regular glucose testing and manage the cost of the extra security that accompanies more continuous testing.

2.9.6 Intake of Fluids

While patients will drink non caloric fluids during intermittent fasting, patients may not understand that except if they drink extra fluids, they are really decreasing their complete liquid admission because of diminished admission of food sources like soups, yogurt, or melons. For this situation, the danger of parchedness and hypotension increments. The patient may then have to decrease or retain their admission of diuretics, SGLT-2 inhibitors, or hostile to hypertensive drugs on the times of fasting.

Chapter 3. Intermittent Fasting Diet plan targets Chronic Inflammation

Analysts say intermittent fasting can lessen irritation in the body. Irritation is one way the body battles contamination, yet on the off chance that there is an excessive amount of aggravation that can prompt different illnesses. Specialists say numerous individuals have an overabundance of irritation since they eat excessively and eat time and again. Intermittent fasting and related weight control plans are having a second. Furthermore, there may be some valid justifications to broaden their 15 minutes of notoriety.

3.1 What is Chronic Inflammation?

Ongoing irritation is additionally alluded to as sluggish, long haul aggravation enduring a while to years. By and large, the degree and impacts of persistent irritation fluctuate with the reason for the injury and the capacity of the body to fix and defeat the harm. This action audits the pathophysiology of ongoing aggravation and features the job of the between proficient group in finding a way to control the pathology. Aggravation is important for the body's safeguard component. It is the interaction by which the invulnerable framework perceives and eliminates hurtful and unfamiliar boosts and starts the mending cycle. Aggravation can be either intense or constant.

Constant irritation is likewise alluded to as sluggish, long haul aggravation going on for delayed times of a while to years. For the most part, the degree and impacts of constant aggravation differ with the reason for the injury and the capacity of the body to fix and defeat the harm. This article audits persistent aggravation.

3.2 Causes of Chronic Inflammation

Disappointment of killing the specialist causing an intense aggravation, for example, irresistible creatures including Mycobacterium tuberculosis, protozoa, organisms, and different parasites that can oppose have safeguards and stay in the tissue for an inclusive period.

Openness to a low level of a specific aggravation or unfamiliar material that can't be disposed of by enzymatic breakdown or phagocytosis in the body including substances or modern synthetic compounds that can be breathed in over a significant stretch, for instance, silica dust.

An immune system issue in which the invulnerable framework perceives the typical part of the body as an unfamiliar antigen, and assaults solid tissue leading to infections like rheumatoid joint pain (RA), foundational lupus erythematosus (SLE).

An imperfection in the cells answerable for interceding irritation prompting relentless or intermittent aggravation, like auto provocative issues (Familial Mediterranean Fever).

Intermittent scenes of intense aggravation. Notwithstanding, at times, persistent irritation is an autonomous reaction and not a spinoff of intense aggravation for instance illnesses like tuberculosis and rheumatoid joint inflammation.

Incendiary and biochemical inducers are causing oxidative pressure and mitochondrial brokenness like expanded creation of free extreme atoms, progressed glycation finished results (AGEs), uric corrosive (urate) gems, oxidized lipoproteins, homocysteine, and others.

3.3 How dangerous is Chronic Inflammation

Ongoing fiery illnesses are the main source of death on the planet. The World Health Organization (WHO) positions ongoing sicknesses as the best danger to human wellbeing. The predominance of illnesses related with ongoing aggravation is expected to increment steadily for the following 30 years in the United States. In 2000, almost 125 million Americans were living with persistent conditions and 61 million (21%) had multiple? In late gauges by Rand Corporation, in 2014 almost 60% of Americans had in any event one constant condition, 42% had multiple and 12% of grownups had at least 5 ongoing conditions. Around the world, 3 of 5 individuals kick the bucket because of ongoing provocative sicknesses like stroke, constant respiratory illnesses, heart issues, malignant growth, stoutness, and diabetes. The predominance of some particular persistent irritation interceded sicknesses are as per the following:

Diabetes: According to the American Diabetes Association, 30.3 million individuals or 9.4% of the American populace, had diabetes in 2015 and it was the seventh driving reason for death in the United States.

Cardiovascular infections: In accordance with 2017 refreshed report from the American Heart Association, cardiovascular sicknesses (CVDs) represents 1 out of each three passing or around 800,000 passing in the United States. Worldwide, CVD represents 31%, everything being equal, and coronary illness (CHD) represents most passing because of CVD, trailed by stroke (1 of 20 passing in the United States) and cardiovascular breakdown.

Joint inflammation and Joint Diseases: These influence around 350 million individuals worldwide and almost 43 million individuals in the United States or practically 20% of the populace. This number is required to surpass 60 million by 2020. Almost, 2.1 million Americans experience the ill effects of rheumatoid joint inflammation.

Sensitivities: These position among the 6th driving reason for ongoing human infections in the United States and influence in excess of 50 million Americans every year. Asthma influences in excess of 24 million individuals in the United States including in excess of 6 million kids. In 2015, 8.2% of grownups and 8.4% of kids were determined to have roughage fever.

Constant Obstructive Pulmonary Disease (COPD): The third most regular reason for death in the United States in 2014, and almost 15.7 million Americans (6.4%) were accounted for to have been determined to have COPD.

3.4 Risk Factors Associated with Chronic Inflammation

Age: Increasing age is decidedly connected with raised levels of a few incendiary particles. The age related expansion in fiery atoms might be expected to mitochondrial brokenness or free extreme gathering over the long haul and other age related variables like an increment in instinctive muscle to fat ratio.

Heftiness: Many examinations have announced that fat tissue is an endocrine organ, discharging various adipokines and other incendiary middle people. A few reports show that the weight list of an individual is relative to the measure of favorable to incendiary cytokines discharged. Metabolic disorder epitomizes this well.

Diet: Diet wealthy in soaked fat, trans fats, or refined sugar is related with higher creation of favorable to fiery atoms, particularly in people with diabetes or overweight people.

Smoking: Cigarette smoking is related with bringing down the creation of calming particles and initiating aggravation.

Low Sex Hormones: Studies show that sex chemicals like testosterone and estrogen can stifle the creation and emission of a few favorable to incendiary markers and it has been seen that keeping up sex chemical levels lessens the danger of a few fiery infections.

Stress and Sleep Disorders: Both physical and enthusiastic pressure is related with fiery cytokine discharge. Stress can likewise cause rest problems. Since people with sporadic rest plans are bound to have persistent irritation than predictable sleepers, rest problems are likewise considered as one of the free danger factors for ongoing aggravation.

3.5 Management of Chronic Inflammation

Numerous dietary and way of life changes might be useful in eliminating irritation triggers and decreasing constant aggravation as recorded underneath. The best is weight reduction. For instance, in patients with psoriatic joint pain which is persistent provocative joint pain, weight reduction alone has been demonstrated to be freely connected with clinically huge improvement in infection movement and irritation.

Low glycemic diet: Diet with a high glycemic file is identified with high danger of stroke, coronary illness, and type 2 diabetes mellitus. It is useful to restrict the utilization of aggravation advancing food sources like soft drinks, refined sugars, and fructose corn syrup in an eating regimen.

Lessen admission of aggregate, soaked fat and trans fats: Some dietary immersed and engineered trans fats exasperate aggravation, while omega-3 polyunsaturated fats seem, by all accounts, to be calming. Prepared and bundled food varieties that contain trans fats like handled seed and vegetable oils, heated products (like soybean and corn oil) ought to be diminished from the eating routine.

Foods grown from the ground: Blueberries, apples, Brussels sprouts, cabbage, broccoli, and cauliflower, that are high in common cancer prevention agents and polyphenols and other calming compounds, may ensure against irritation. Cherries and cherry juice utilization has been demonstrated to be uricosuric and inhibitory for IL-1 in patients with gout.

Fiber: High admission of dietary solvent and insoluble fiber is related with bringing down degrees of IL-6 and TNF-alpha.

Nuts, for example, almonds are related with bringing down the danger of cardiovascular infection and diabetes.

Green and dark tea polyphenols: Tea polyphenols are related with a decrease in CRP in human clinical examinations.

Curcumin: a constituent of turmeric has been demonstrated to be related with critical improvement in a few incendiary sicknesses in creature models.

Fish Oil: The most extravagant wellspring of the omega-3 unsaturated fats. Higher admission of omega-3 unsaturated fats is related with bringing down degrees of TNF-alpha, CRP, and IL-6.

Mung bean: Rich in flavonoids (especially vitexin and isovitexin). It is a conventional food and home grown medication known for its mitigating impacts.

Micronutrients: Magnesium, nutrient D, nutrient E, zinc and selenium). Magnesium is recorded as quite possibly the most mitigating dietary variables, and its admission is related with the bringing down of hsCRP, IL-6, and TNF-alpha movement. Nutrient D applies its calming action by smothering incendiary go between, for example, prostaglandins and atomic factor kappa light chain enhancer of enacted B cells. Nutrient E, zinc, and selenium go about as cancer prevention agents in the body.

Sesame Lignans: Sesame oil utilization diminishes the blend of prostaglandin, leukotrienes, and thromboxanes and is known for its expected hypotensive action.

3.6 Diet and Inflammation

The examination discoveries answer how that association among diet and aggravation works. However, the exercises that eating less can diminish irritation and issues related with it aren't new. We're reliably over powering, and that at that point prompts what I would call fiery pathways. So time confined eating limits that. Saying this doesn't imply that that food isn't significant. It's just about control.

One thing that prescribed to a portion of the customers is to just eat between specific hours of the day just as staying away from sugars. It is recommended just eating between 11 a.m. also, 7 p.m. for instance, which to some degree imitates circadian rhythms. This time limited eating has been appeared to improve in general gut wellbeing and miniature biota, which immensely affects wellbeing.

How does a calming count calories respond? Your insusceptible framework becomes actuated when your body remembers whatever is unfamiliar like an attacking organism, plant dust, or synthetic. This regularly triggers an interaction called irritation. Discontinuous episodes of irritation coordinated at genuinely compromising trespassers secure your wellbeing.

Notwithstanding, now and again aggravation continues, all day every day, in any event, when you are not undermined by an unfamiliar intruder. That is when irritation can turn into your foe. Many significant sicknesses that plague us including malignancy, coronary illness, diabetes, joint pain, sorrow, and Alzheimer's have been connected to constant aggravation.

Quite possibly the most integral assets to battle aggravation comes not from the drug store, but rather from the supermarket. "Numerous test contemplates have shown that segments of food sources or drinks may have calming impacts.

Pick the correct calming food varieties, and you might have the option to lessen your danger of sickness. Reliably pick some unacceptable ones, and you could speed up the provocative illness measure.

Of course, similar food varieties on an irritation diet are for the most part thought to be awful for our wellbeing, including soft drinks and refined sugars, just as red meat and handled meats.

A portion of the food varieties that have been related with an expanded danger for persistent illnesses, for example, type 2 diabetes and coronary illness are likewise connected with abundance irritation. It's to be expected, since aggravation is a significant basic instrument for the advancement of these illnesses.

Unfortunate food sources additionally add to weight acquire, which is itself a danger factor for irritation. However in a few examinations, even after analysts considered corpulence, the connection among food varieties and irritation remained, which recommends weight acquire isn't the sole driver. A portion of the food segments or fixings may affect irritation well beyond expanded caloric admission.

On the other side are refreshments and food varieties that diminish aggravation, and with it, constant sickness, says Dr. Hu. He notes specifically foods grown from the ground like blueberries, apples, and mixed greens that are high in regular cancer prevention agents and polyphenols defensive mixtures found in plants.

Studies have additionally connected nuts with decreased markers of aggravation and a lower hazard of cardiovascular illness and diabetes. Espresso, which contains polyphenols and other calming compounds, may ensure against irritation, also.

To lessen levels of irritation, focus on a generally sound eating routine. In case you're searching for an eating plan that intently follows the fundamentals of calming eating, think about the Mediterranean eating regimen, which is high in natural products, vegetables, nuts, entire grains, fish, and solid oils.

As well as bringing down irritation, a more common, less handled eating routine can effectsly affect your physical and passionate wellbeing. A solid eating routine is gainful not just for decreasing the danger of persistent infections, yet in addition for improving disposition and by and large personal satisfaction.

3.7 What Researchers Discovered

In the new investigation, the human members accomplished something somewhat unique. They weren't permitted to eat among early afternoon and 3 p.m. right off the bat, and afterward not between 8 p.m. that very day until 3 p.m. of the next day. They were permitted to drink water. At 3 p.m. on the two days, blood was attracted to test white platelet levels. White platelets, of which monocytes are one sort, are the body's insurance against contamination and normally show aggravation.

Another investigation has inferred that intermittent fasting decreases irritation, a condition that can prompt different illnesses like diabetes, various sclerosis, and fiery inside disorder. That decrease, the examination found, was because of a decrease in cells that cause irritation called "monocytes" in the blood.

Analysts likewise said the monocytes that were in the blood were less incendiary than they were in individuals and mice not on intermittent fasting diet. The justification the distinction might be less that it's acceptable to starve yourself as that every other person is eating excessively. Particularly in the Western world, individuals eat constantly and that is a genuinely ongoing propensity in human advancement.

Aggravation is a helpful instrument our bodies use to battle contaminations. Be that as it may, the amount of irritation causing cells we regularly have today might be more a result of this indulging than need. We puzzled over whether the quantity of monocytes we call typical is, indeed, not ordinary truth be told puts us in danger and might be pointless, may mirror our new dietary propensities, some way or another we have obtained dietary propensities that are putting us in danger for aggravation.

We use them to realize whether somebody is wiped out and there are numbers that are viewed as ordinary. Individuals with a contamination have enormous numbers. What we saw here is an exceptionally solid drop in monocytes. A recent report inferred that fasting for over 24 hours may bring down irritation by decreasing oxidative pressure in cells. A recent report tracked down that both intermittent fasting and substitute day fasting were pretty much as powerful as restricting calorie consumption at lessening insulin obstruction.

In any case, it is expected to look further into changed weight control plans including into any potential adverse consequences they may have. And afterward we will truly begin to comprehend whether we can disclose solid proposals to the.

Not at all like eating regimens that cut out or down on specific food sources, intermittent fasting normally includes simply not eating at specific occasions. Regularly, that implies refraining for 16 to 24 hours, typically double seven days. At its generally outrageous, individuals will cease from nourishment for 48 hours. Intermittent fasting is turning out to be truly chic, however a few group are doing insane things like not eating for quite a long time. Yet, the fact isn't to quit eating. What I'm saying is we most likely eat excessively and again and again certainly we eat time after time.

Analysts have tracked down that a compound delivered by the body when counting calories or fasting can obstruct a piece of the insusceptible framework associated with a few fiery problems, for example, type 2 diabetes, atherosclerosis, and Alzheimer's illness.

In their examination, distributed in the Feb. 16 online issue of Nature Medicine, the analysts portrayed how the compound beta hydroxybutyrate (BHB) straightforwardly represses NLRP3, which is essential for an intricate arrangement of proteins called the inflammasome. The inflammasome drives the provocative reaction in a few issues including immune system sicknesses, type 2 diabetes, atherosclerosis, Alzheimer's infection and auto fiery issues.

These discoveries are significant on the grounds that endogenous metabolites like BHB that block the NLRP3 inflammasome could be pertinent against numerous provocative sicknesses, remembering those where there are changes for the NLRP3 qualities.

BHB is a metabolite delivered by the body in light of fasting, focused energy work out, caloric limitation, or utilization of the low sugar ketogenic diet. Dixit said it is notable that fasting and calorie limitation lessens irritation in the body, yet it was muddled how safe cells adjust to diminished accessibility of glucose and on the off chance that they can react to metabolites delivered from fat oxidation.

Working with mice and human insusceptible cells, additionally centered on how macrophages specific safe cells that produce irritation react when presented to ketone bodies and whether that impacts the inflammasone complex.

The group acquainted BHB with mouse models of provocative sicknesses brought about by NLP3. They tracked down that this diminished irritation, and that aggravation was likewise decreased when the mice were given a ketogenic diet, which hoists the degrees of BHB in the circulatory system.

Our outcomes propose that the endogenous metabolites like BHB that are created during low carb slimming down, fasting, or extreme focus exercise can bring down the NLRP3 inflammasome.

3.8 Anti-inflammatory Mechanism of Intermittent Fasting Diet Plan

Intermittent fasting is known as a craze, yet it is a custom that has been seen by societies all throughout the planet for centuries. Various investigations have discovered potential medical advantages (and outcomes) related with fasting, the idea of which relies upon the kind of quick. Though certain fasting conventions require an individual to burn through just water for various hours or days, others permit organic product juice or enormously limited food utilization.

In present day times, fasting is frequently embraced with an end goal to initiate autophagy, a cycle by which the body clears out old harmed cells and replaces them with fresher and better cells. It's muddled how long a human should quick for autophagy to be initiated, yet many accept that at any rate 24 hours is essential to get this advantage.

Not every person can quick for that long of a period, notwithstanding, prompting the ascent of intermittent fasting, a kind of fasting convention that ordinarily includes swearing off nourishment for a specific number of hours in a day. Somebody who diets may just burn through water, and conceivably tea or espresso, for 18 hours, as one model, with the excess six hours of the day being the time span during which food can be devoured.

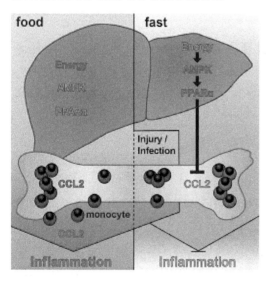

Intermittent fasting conventions that last under 24 hours may have a valuable impact for people experiencing constant irritation, another investigation as of late distributed in Cell has found. The exploration emerges from Mount Sinai, where researchers tracked down that intermittent fasting decreases the quantity of monocytes circling in the blood.

These cells are favorable to fiery; significant levels are available in instances of immune system sicknesses and certain different conditions. Intense that is, brief snapshots of aggravation is a typical and essential cycle set off by the safe framework to dispose of diseases. Notwithstanding, persistent aggravation the sort that goes on for significant stretches of time can prompt countless wellbeing outcomes, including the improvement of malignant growth, coronary illness, and the sky is the limit from there.

The investigation tracked down that intermittent fasting diminishes the resistant framework's irritation reaction and prompts enhancements in illnesses including ongoing aggravation, yet it does this without trading off the body's capacity to target contaminations.

Intermittent fasting is possibly hazardous in certain people, especially on the off chance that one diets for an extensive stretch of time. Anybody considering fasting under any circumstance should converse with their PCP first to ensure their body can deal with the slimming down convention.

Intermittent fasting regimens have acquired public and logical interest as of late, however fasting shouldn't be excused as a trend. In an investigation distributed, analysts found that fasting decreases aggravation and improves persistent provocative illnesses without influencing the invulnerable framework's reaction to intense contaminations.

While intense irritation is an ordinary insusceptible interaction that assists battle with offing contaminations, constant aggravation can have genuine ramifications for wellbeing, including coronary illness, diabetes, malignancy, numerous sclerosis, and fiery gut infections.

Caloric limitation is known to improve fiery and immune system infections, yet the components by which diminished caloric admission controls irritation have been inadequately perceived, said an analyst.

Working with human insusceptible cells, analyst showed that intermittent fasting decreased the arrival of favorable to fiery cells called "monocytes" in blood course. Further examinations uncovered that during times of fasting, these phones go into "rest mode" and are less incendiary than monocytes found in the individuals who were taken care of.

Monocytes are profoundly provocative invulnerable cells that can cause genuine tissue harm, and the populace has seen an expanding sum in their blood course because of dietary patterns that people have procured in ongoing hundreds of years. Considering the expansive range of illnesses that are brought about by constant irritation and the expanding number of patients influenced by these infections, there is a huge potential in researching the mitigating impacts of fasting.

Scientists intend to keep attempting to interpret the subatomic instruments by which fasting improves incendiary sicknesses, which could prompt novel preventive restorative methodologies for the therapy of numerous human infections.

Conclusion

Intermittent fasting, when embraced for wellbeing reasons in patients with diabetes mellitus, the two kinds 1 and 2, has been appeared in a couple of little human examinations to prompt weight reduction and diminish insulin necessities. While these discoveries are energizing and have caught the creative mind of numerous individuals, an astute way to deal with executing fasting regimens and utilizing them in the long haul among this particular populace is required. A significant part of the promotion encompassing fasting emerges from creature examines, which just propose what human exploration ought to be directed; execution of human intercessions ought not to be founded on creature research.

Long haul advantages of fasting, including cardiovascular danger decrease, stay to be completely considered and clarified, particularly in people. Clinicians should temper the eagerness for fasting with the truth that the advantages and dangers in people remain to a great extent neglected and the advantages may require a long time to years to show up or be completely figured it out. Great proof from epidemiologic investigations, pilot interventional preliminaries, and a couple of randomized preliminaries recommends that the advantages of fasting exceed the likely damages in the normal person. Individuals with diabetes, be that as it may, are not the normal individual, and their own necessities require more cautious thought toward the start of and during the utilization of a fasting routine. With legitimate drug change and observing of blood glucose levels however, intermittent fasting can be supported and securely executed among individuals with diabetes.

Lightning Source UK Ltd.
Milton Keynes UK
UKHW020642270521
384471UK00010B/739